KEIRA COLLINS

KETO

SLOW COOKER

RECIPES

COOKBOOK

The Ultimate Healthy Low-Carb Recipe Guide to Succeed on Your Keto Diet Without Compromising on Taste

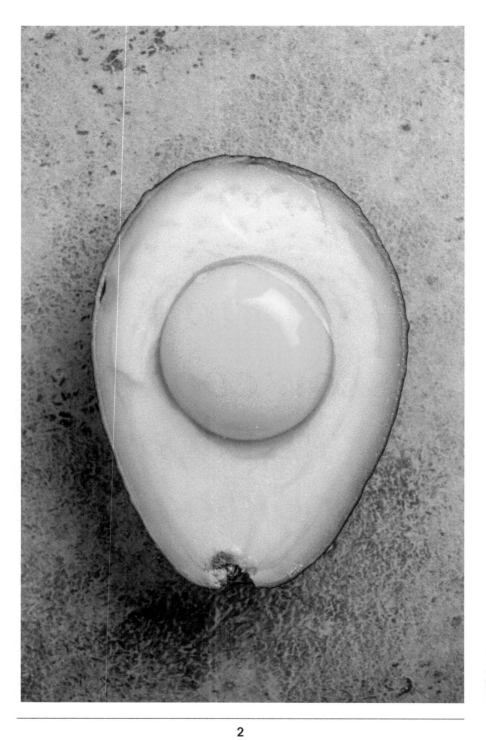

Table of Contents

Food to Eat & Food to Avoid

Food to Eat

- Grass-fed and wild animal meat:

    Grass-fed meat such as goat, lamb, beef, seafood, and wild-caught fish. Eat high in Omega 3 fatty acid from pastured eggs, butter, gelatin, pastured poultry, and pork. Eat grass-fed organs meat such as liver, kidneys, and hearts.

- Healthy Fats:

    Add some healthy fats to daily diet plans such as fats and their sources given below

- Saturated fats:

    These fats are found in goose fat, duck fat, coconut oil, butter, tallow, chicken fat, and lard.

- Polyunsaturated fats:

    These fats are found from animal sources such as seafood and fatty fish; it contains Omega 3 fatty acids.

- Monounsaturated fats:

    Mainly get this fat from olive oil, avocado oil, and macadamia oil.

- Fruits and non-starchy vegetables:

- Fruits:

    Avocado is the only fruit suitable for the keto diet.

- Non-Starchy Vegetables:

    Green and leafy vegetables such as spinach, chard, endive, bok choy, radicchio, lettuce.

Also use cruciferous vegetables like radishes, kohlrabi, kale, etc.

Cucumber, asparagus, bamboo shoots, celery stalk are used in ketogenic diet meals.

- Condiments and beverages:
- Black or herbal tea, black coffee, cream coffee, water.
- Fermented foods such as kombucha, kimchi, and sauerkraut, mayonnaise, pesto, bone broth, mustard, and pickles.
- All herbs and spices are used such as lime juice and zest

Eat Occasionally

- Fruits vegetables and mushroom:
- Cruciferous vegetables such as all cabbages, broccoli, cauliflower, fennel, Brussel sprouts, etc.
- Sea vegetables such as sugar snap peas, French artichokes, okra, bean sprouts, and wax beans.
- Root vegetables such as onion, mushrooms, pumpkin, leek, and garlic.
- Berries such as blue barriers, blackberries, cranberries, strawberries, raspberries, mulberries, etc.
- Full Fat Dairy products:
- Dairy products such as cottage cheese, full-fat yogurt, sour cream, heavy cream, etc.
- Nuts and seeds:
- Pine nuts, pumpkin seeds, walnut, pecans, sunflower seeds, sesame seeds, hemp seeds, almonds
- Macadamia nuts are high in monounsaturated fats and it has a very low carb
- Fermented soy products:
- Eat fermented soy products such as tamari, natto, tempeh

- Unprocessed green and black soybeans
- Alcohol:
- Unsweetened spirits, dry white wine, and dry red wine.

Food to Avoid

- Processed Food: Avoid processed food that contains carrageen as sulfites gelatin and dried fruits, MSG found in some whey protein products, wheat gluten, etc.
- All grains: Whole grains such as oats, wheat, millet, sprouted grains, rice, buckwheat, millet, bulgur, sorghum.
- All products are made from grains such as pizza, cookies, pasta, crackers, bread, etc. sweets and sugar such as agave syrup, cakes, ice cream soft drinks, and sweet puddings.
- Artificial sweeteners: Avoid artificial sweeteners because they cause carving which produces some health issues such as migraines such as Splenda, equal, and sweeteners which contain Aspartame, sucralose, acesulfame, etc.
- Food with added sugar: Avoid sweeteners that raise your blood sugar, these cause insulin spikes.
- Refined oils: Canola, cottonseeds, soybean, sunflower, safflower, corn, grape seed oils.
- Tropical fruits: Such as mango, banana, pineapple, papaya, etc. avoid some high carb fruits like grapes, tangerine. Also avoid fresh fruit juices, dried fruits like raisins, dates.
- Legumes: Legumes are high in the carb so avoid legumes. It is also hard to digest due to they contain phytates and lectins.
- Avoid soy products: Avoid soy products except for a few non-GMO fermented products which have health benefits and also avoid wheat gluten and use BPA-free packaging.
- Milk: Milk is not easily digested. Less number of good bacteria is present in milk. You may take a small amount of raw milk.

- Alcoholic, sweet drinks: Beer, cocktails, sweet wine, etc. You can consume low carb drinks and cocktails

Tips

1. Only consumes keto food and ingredients
2. Track your daily calories intake
3. Plan your meals ahead of times
4. Avoid convenient food
5. Eat those foods that you measure and track
6. Use the meal plan which helps you keep track of your calories
7. Always meal preparation for the week
8. Make your drinks keto-friendly
9. While following the keto diet pair a workout with it
10. Consume good fats which provide omega 3
11. Drink lots of water if you follow weight loss
12. To make your favorite meal use low carb ingredients
13. Avoid sugar carving using herbs
14. Keep your energy up with juice and teas
15. Always eat healthy fats
16. Don't over-consume protein
17. You have to moderate your protein intake
18. Do not compromise your food quality

FAQS

Where can I find low carb keto recipes?

- Everywhere on the internet. You can find low carb recipes on health and nutrition websites.

How should I track my carb intake?

- There are various ways to measure carb intake. One of the most common is a mobile fitness app that helps to keep track.

Can I eat too much fat?

- Eating too much fat will push over calories deficit and convert it into a calorie.

Can I drink alcohol during the diet?

- Yes, alcohol can be consumed during a diet but be careful about hidden carbs in the drink.

How long does it take to get ketosis?

- If you are in your optimal carb limit usually it will take 2-3 days to enter ketosis.

Can I eat nuts?

- You can eat nuts but in moderation. Nuts are suitable for a ketogenic diet.

Can I eat fruits?

- Yes, you can eat avocados and coconut. You can also eat a moderate amount of low carb fruits such as berries.

Is a ketogenic diet suitable for kids?

- Yes, the ketosis diet is widely used to cure diseases like autism and epilepsy in kids.

Breakfast

French Omelet

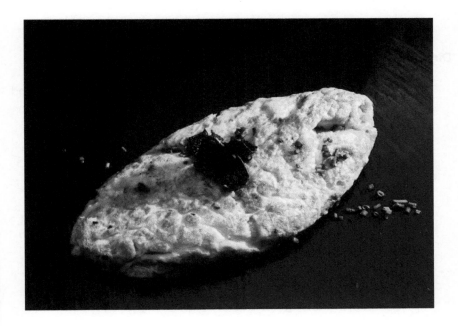

Preparation Time: 10 minutes

Cooking Time: 1 hour

Servings: 2

Ingredients:

- 4 eggs

- Salt to taste

- Pepper to taste

- ⅔ cup Swiss cheese, grated

- 1 tbsp. butter, melted

- 2 tbsp. half and half or milk

- 2 tbsp. sour cream + a little to garnish

- ⅔ cup sautéed spinach, drained

- 2 strips lemon peel

Directions:

1. Whisk together in a bowl, eggs, half and half, sour cream, salt, and pepper.

2. Add butter into the slow cooker. Swirl the pot so that the butter coats the bottom of the pot. Pour the beaten egg mixture into it.

3. Close the lid. Select 'High' and set the timer for 20-30 minutes or 'Low' for 45-60 minutes. Cook until the omelet is very soft and set.

4. Place spinach and cheese on one half of the omelet. Fold the other part over it.

5. Serve immediately garnished with lemon strip and sour cream.

Nutrition:

- Calories 382.1

- Carbohydrate 4.2 g

- Protein 23.4 g

- Fat 30 g

- Sugar: 0.9 g

- Sodium: 1123 mg

- Fiber: 3.4 g

Healthy Slow Cooker Frittata

Preparation Time: 10 minutes

Cooking Time: 1 hour

Servings: 8

Ingredients:

- 12 large eggs, beaten
- 1 ½ cups artichoke hearts, chopped
- ½ cup yellow bell pepper, chopped
- ½ cup low-fat cheddar cheese, grated
- Salt to taste
- Pepper to taste
- 1 tomato, deseeded, chopped
- ½ cup green onion, chopped
- Cooking spray

Directions:

1. Spray the bottom of the slow cooker with cooking spray.
2. Add all the ingredients except cheese into a bowl and mix well.
3. Pour into the slow cooker.
4. Close the lid. Select 'Low' and set the timer for 1-2 hours or until well set.
5. Sprinkle cheese on top. Cover and let it sit for some time.

6. Chop into 8 wedges and serve. Leftovers can be stored in an airtight container in the refrigerator.

Nutrition:

- Calories: 141

- Carbohydrate: 3 g

- Protein: 12 g

- Fat: 9 g

- Sugar: 1.4 g

- Sodium: 1723 mg

- Fiber: 5.9 g

Egg and Cottage Cheese Savory Breakfast

Muffins

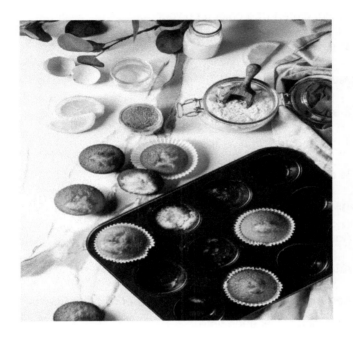

Preparation Time: 10 minutes

Cooking Time: 2 hours

Servings: 6

Ingredients:

Dry Ingredients:

- ¼ cup almond meal

- ¼ cup parmesan cheese, finely grated

- 2 tbsp. nutritional yeast flakes

- ¼ tsp. spike seasoning (optional)

- ¼ cup raw hemp seeds

- 2 tbsp. flaxseed meal

- ¼ tsp. gluten-free baking powder

- ⅛ tsp. salt or to taste

Wet Ingredients:

- 3 eggs, beaten

- 1 green onion, thinly sliced

- ¼ cup low fat cottage cheese

Directions:

1. Add all the dry ingredients into a bowl and mix until well combined.

2. Add all the wet ingredients into a large bowl and whisk well.

3. Add the dry ingredients into the bowl of wet ingredients, a little at a time, and whisk each time.

4. When all the dry ingredients are added, spoon into greased muffin molds. Fill up to ¾ the mold.

5. Place crumpled aluminum foil at the bottom of the cooker (this step can be avoided if your cooking pot is ceramic).

6. Place the muffin molds inside the cooker.

7. Close the lid. Set cooker on 'High' option and timer for 2-3 hours. Check after 2 hours of cooking. If it is not looking done, then cook for some more time.

8. If you like the top to be dry, then uncover and cook during the last 40-60 minutes of cooking.

9. For the medium top, you can place a chopstick on the top of the cooker before closing the lid.

10. Let it cool in the cooker for a while.

11. Cool slightly. Run a knife around the edges. Serve on a plate and serve immediately.

Nutrition:

- Calories: 143

- Carbohydrate: 6 g

- Protein: 9 g

- Fat: 10 g Sugar: 4.4 g Sodium: 1133 mg

- Fiber: 6.9 g

Broccoli and Sausage Casserole

Preparation Time: 10 minutes

Cooking Time: 5 hour

Servings: 3

Ingredients:

- 1 small head broccoli, chopped

- ½ cup cheddar cheese, shredded

- 6 tbsp. whipping cream

- ¼ tsp. salt or to taste

- Pepper to taste

- 6 oz. Jones Dairy farm little links (breakfast sausage) cooked, sliced

- 5 eggs

- 1 clove garlic, minced

- Cooking spray

Directions:

1. Spray the inside of the slow cooker with cooking spray. Be generous with the spray.

2. Spread the broccoli at the bottom of the pot. Layer with sausage slices all over the broccoli followed by cheese.

3. Whisk together in a bowl, eggs, whipping cream, pepper, salt, and garlic. Pour into the slow cooker.

4. Close the lid. Select the 'Low' option and timer for 4-5 hours or on the 'High' option and timer for 2-3 hours or until the edges are brown and it is not jiggling in the center.

5. Serve hot or warm.

Nutrition:

- Calories: 484

- Carbohydrates: 5.39 g

- Protein: 26.13g

- Fat: 38.86 g

- Sugar: 2.4 g

- Sodium: 1343 mg

- Fiber: 4.0 g

Lunch Recipes

Mediterranean Turkey Roast

Preparation Time: 20 minutes

Cooking Time: 7 hours and 30 minutes

Servings: 4

Ingredients:

- 2 lbs. turkey breast boneless, trimmed

- 1 cup onion chopped

- ¼ cup oil-packed sun-dried tomatoes chopped

- ¼ cup Kalamata olives pitted

- 1 tsp. garlic minced

- 1 tbsp. fresh lemon juice

- ½ tsp. Greek seasoning mix

- ¼ tsp. salt

- Ground pepper to taste

- ¼ cup chicken broth divided

- 2 tbsp. coconut or almond flour

- 2 tbsp. butter

- A few sprigs thyme

Directions:

1. Except for the flour and half of the chicken broth, add all the ingredients to the Crock-Pot.

2. Cover and cook on low for 7 hours.

3. Mix together the flour and remaining broth and pour into the pot.

4. Mix well and cook on low for 30 minutes more.

5. Chop the turkey into slices and serve.

Nutrition:

- Calories: 336

- Carbs: 14.3 g

- Protein: 43.2 g

- Fat: 11.2 g

- Sugar: 5.3 g

- Sodium: 1522 mg

- Fiber: 8.9 g

Rump Roast

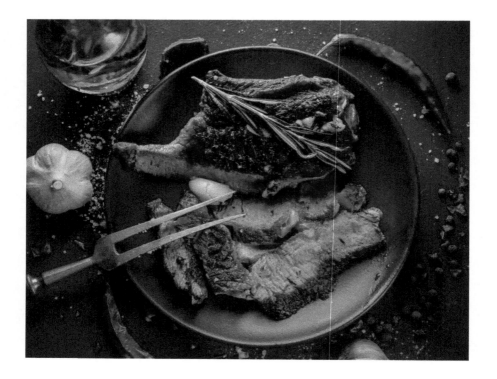

Preparation Time: 20 minutes

Cooking Time: 10 hours

Servings: 4

Ingredients:

- 1 (3 lbs.) rump roast

- 1 onion diced

- 1 tbsp. black pepper

- 1 tbsp. paprika

- 2 tbsp. chili powder

- ½ tsp. cayenne

- ½ tsp. garlic

- ¼ tsp. mustard powder

- ½ cup beef stock

- ⅓ cup butter

Directions:

1. Combine all the spices and mix well. Generously rub the spice mixture all over the rump roast. Then rub with butter.

2. Line the bottom of the Crock-Pot with diced onions.

3. Place seasoned roast on top. Pour in the beef stock.

4. Cover and cook on low for 10 hours.

Nutrition:

- Calories: 514

- Carbs: 5.6 g

- Protein: 58.1 g

- Fat: 29 g

- Sugar: 5.3 g

- Sodium: 1522 mg

- Fiber: 8.9 g

Herb Chicken

Preparation Time: 20 minutes

Cooking time: 3 hours and 35 minutes

Servings: 4 to 6

Ingredients:

- 1 whole chicken cut-up
- 1 large onion cut into thin slices
- 1 tbsp. garlic chopped
- 1 ½ tsp. thyme
- 1 tsp. basil leaves
- 1 tsp. oregano leaves
- 1 tsp. salt
- ½ tsp. pepper
- 2 tbsp. olive oil

Directions:

1. Grease the Crock-Pot with oil. Add onion.
2. Mix the oregano, thyme, salt, basil, garlic, and pepper in a bowl. Rub the chicken pieces with the mixture.
3. Place the chicken in the Crock-Pot in a single layer.
4. Cover and cook on high for 3 ½ hours.

5. Set your oven to broil.

6. Remove the chicken from the Crock-Pot and place (skin side up) on a broiler pan lined with foil.

7. Broil with tops 6 inches from the heat. Broil for 5 to 6 minutes or until chicken is golden brown.

Nutrition:

- Calories: 550

- Carbs: 3 g

- Protein: 85 g

- Fat: 22 g

- Sugar: 5.3 g

- Sodium: 1522 mg

- Fiber: 8.9 g

Beef Lasagna

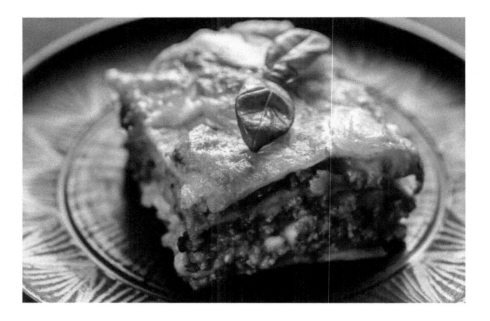

Preparation Time: 20 minutes

Cooking Time: 4 hours

Servings: 4

Ingredients:

- 1 lb. minced beef

- ½ onion finely chopped

- 3 garlic cloves chopped

- 1 tsp. dried mixed herbs (oregano, rosemary, thyme)

- ½ eggplant cut into slices

- 1 large zucchini cut into slices

- 1 cup baby spinach

- 1 cup grated cheddar cheese

- 2 tomatoes chopped

- ½ cup grated mozzarella cheese

- ½ cup ricotta cheese

- 4 tbsp. olive oil

Directions:

1. Heat half of the oil in a pan and sauté onions and garlic until onions are soft.

2. Add the minced beef to the pan and cook for 3 minutes to brown.

3. Add the tomatoes and mixed herbs to the beef and sprinkle with salt and pepper. Cook for 5 minutes.

4. Add the rest of the oil into the Crock-Pot.

5. Spread a layer of beef mixture into the pot.

6. Place a layer of eggplant over the beef.

7. Add another thin layer of beef mixture over the eggplant.

8. Place a layer of zucchini over the beef.

9. Add another layer of beef over the zucchini.

10. Place the spinach leaves over the beef.

11. Add the remaining beef mixture over the spinach.

12. In a large bowl, mix together the cheddar cheese, mozzarella, ricotta, salt, and pepper.

13. Spread the cheese mixture over the lasagna.

14. Cover with the lid and cook on high for 4 hours.

15. Serve.

Nutrition:

- Calories: 391

- Carbs: 12.8 g

- Protein: 35.2 g

- Fat: 23.1 g

- Sugar: 5.3 g

- Sodium: 1522 mg

- Fiber: 8.9 g

Dinner Recipes

Beef and Broccoli

Preparation Time: 5 minutes

Cooking Time: 25 minutes

Servings: 4

Ingredients:

- 1 ½ lb. chuck roast, sliced

- 12 oz. broccoli florets

- 4 garlic cloves peeled

- 2 tbsp. avocado oil

- ½ cup soy sauce

- ¼ cup Erythritol sweetener

- 1 tbsp. Xanthan gum

Directions:

1. Switch on the instant pot, grease the pot with oil, press the 'sauté/simmer' button, wait until the oil is hot and add the beef slices and garlic and cook for 5 to 10 minutes or until browned.

2. Meanwhile, whisk together sweetener, soy sauce, and broth until combined.

3. Pour sauce over browned beef, toss until well coated, then press the 'keep warm' button and shut the instant pot with its lid in the sealed position.

4. Press the 'manual' button, press '+/-' to set the cooking time to 10 minutes, and cook at a high-pressure setting; when the pressure builds in the pot, the cooking timer will start.

5. Meanwhile, place broccoli florets in a large heatproof bowl, cover with plastic wrap, and microwave for 4 minutes or until tender.

6. When the instant pot buzzes, press the 'keep warm' button, do a quick pressure release and open the lid.

7. Take out ¼ cup of cooking liquid, stir in xanthan gum until combined, then add into the instant pot and stir until mixed.

8. Press the 'sauté/simmer' button and simmer beef and sauce for 5 minutes or until the sauce reaches the desired consistency.

9. Then add broccoli florets, stir until mixed and press the cancel button.

10. Serve broccoli and beef with cauliflower rice.

Nutrition:

- Calories: 351.4
- Fat: 12.4 g
- Protein: 29 g
- Carbs: 11 g
- Fiber: 8 g
- Total Fat: 23 g
- Saturated Fat: 10 g
- Sugar: 2 g

Korean Barbecue Beef

Preparation Time: 5 minutes

Cooking Time: 25 minutes

Servings: 4

Ingredients:

- 3 lb. beef chuck roast, fat trimmed, cubed

- ½ cup beef broth

- ⅓ cup Erythritol sweetener

- ¼ cup liquid aminos

- 2 tbsp. minced garlic

- 2 tbsp. avocado oil

- 1 tbsp. apple cider vinegar

- 1 tbsp. grated ginger

- 1 ½ tsp. Sriracha sauce

- ½ tsp. ground black pepper tsp.

Directions:

1. Switch on the instant pot, add all the ingredients, and stir until mixed.

2. Shut the instant pot with its lid in the sealed position, then press the 'manual' button, press '+/-' to set the cooking time to 25 minutes, and cook at a high-pressure setting; when the pressure builds in the pot, the cooking timer will start.

3. When the instant pot buzzes, press the 'keep warm' button, release pressure naturally for 10 minutes, then do a quick pressure release and open the lid.

4. Garnish beef with cilantro and serve.

Nutrition:

- Calories: 635.7
- Fat: 31.7 g
- Protein: 69.3 g
- Carbs: 10.5 g
- Total Fat: 23 g
- Saturated Fat: 10 g
- Sugar: 2 g
- Fiber: 17.3 g

Whole Chicken

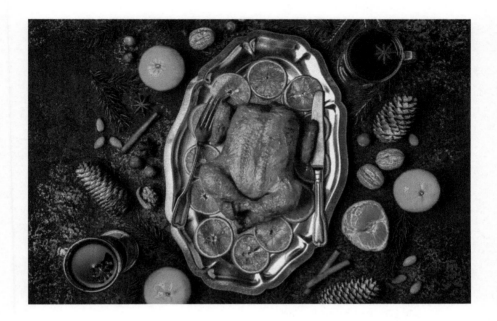

Preparation Time: 5 minutes

Cooking Time: 25 minutes

Servings: 7

Ingredients:

- 5 lb. medium whole chicken

- 1 ½ tsp. minced garlic

- 1 tbsp. avocado oil

- ⅛ tsp. sea salt

- ¼ tsp. ground black pepper

- 1 lemon sliced

- 2 cups water

- 1 tbsp. apple cider vinegar

Directions:

1. Brush chicken with oil, then rub with salt and black pepper and stuff its cavity with lemon slices.

2. Switch on the instant pot, pour in water, add vinegar, then place the chicken on it and shut the instant pot with its lid in the sealed position.

3. Press the 'manual' button, press '+/-' to set the cooking time to 25 minutes, and cook at a high-pressure setting; when the pressure builds in the pot, the cooking timer will start.

4. When the instant pot buzzes, press the 'keep warm' button, release pressure naturally for 10 minutes, then do a quick pressure release and open the lid.

5. Transfer chicken to a cutting board, let it rest for 10 minutes, then cut into pieces and serve.

Nutrition:

- Calories: 209
- Fat: 5 g
- Protein: 41 g
- Carbs: 1 g
- Total Fat: 23 g
- Saturated Fat: 10 g
- Sugar: 2 g
- Fiber: 0 g

Garlic Chicken

Preparation Time: 5 minutes

Cooking Time: 35 minutes

Servings: 4

Ingredients:

- 4 chicken breasts
- 1 tsp. salt
- ¼ cup avocado oil
- 1 tsp. turmeric powder
- 10 cloves garlic, peeled and diced

Directions:

1. Switch on the instant pot, add chicken, then season with salt and black pepper, pour in the oil, and scatter garlic on top.

2. Shut the instant pot with its lid in the sealed position, then press the 'manual' button, press '+/-' to set the cooking time to 35 minutes, and cook at a high-pressure setting; when the pressure builds in the pot, the cooking timer will start.

3. When the instant pot buzzes, press the 'keep warm' button, release pressure naturally for 10 minutes, then do a quick pressure release and open the lid.

4. Shred chicken with two forks, toss until mixed and serve as a lettuce wrap.

Nutrition:

- Calories: 404

- Fat: 21 g

- Protein: 47 g

- Carbs: 3 g

- Total Fat: 23 g

- Saturated Fat: 10 g

- Sugar: 2 g

- Fiber: 0 g

Appetizers & Snacks

Radish Spinach Medley

Preparation Time: 10 minutes

Cooking Time: 2 hours

Servings: 2

Ingredients:

- 1 lb. spinach, torn

- 2 cups radishes, sliced

- A pinch salt and black pepper

- ¼ cup vegetable broth

- 1 tsp. chili powder

- 1 tbsp. parsley, chopped

Directions:

1. Start by throwing all the ingredients into the Crock-Pot.

2. Cover its lid and cook for 2 hours on a low setting.

3. Once done, remove its lid of the Crock-Pot carefully.

4. Mix well and garnish as desired.

5. Serve warm.

Nutrition:

- Calories: 244
- Total Fat: 24.8 g
- Saturated Fat: 15.6 g
- Cholesterol: 32 mg
- Sodium: 204 mg
- Total Carbs: 2.1 g
- Sugar: 0.4 g
- Fiber: 0.1 g
- Protein: 24 g

Citrus rich Cabbage

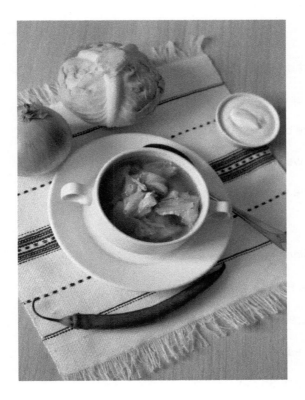

Preparation Time: 10 minutes

Cooking Time: 3 hours

Servings: 2

Ingredients:

- 1 lb. green cabbage, shredded

- ½ cup chicken stock

- A pinch salt and black pepper

- 1 tbsp. lemon juice

- 1 tbsp. chives, diced

- 1 tbsp. lemon zest (grated)

Directions:

1. Start by throwing all the ingredients into the Crock-Pot.

2. Cover its lid and cook for 3 hours on a low setting.

3. Once done, remove its lid of the Crock-Pot carefully.

4. Mix well and garnish as desired.

5. Serve warm.

Nutrition:

- Calories: 145

- Total Fat: 13.1 g

- Saturated Fat: 9.1 g

- Cholesterol: 96 mg

- Sodium: 35 mg

- Total Carbs: 4 g

- Sugar: 1.2 g

- Fiber: 1.5 g

- Protein: 3.5 g

Spiced Lemon Drink

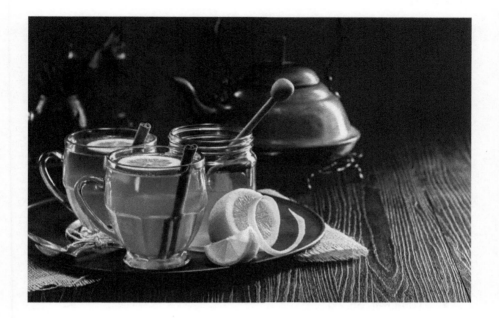

Preparation Time: 10 minutes

Cooking Time: 3 hours

Servings: 4

Ingredients:

- 2½ quarts water
- 2 cups stevia
- 1½ cups lime juice
- ½ cup plus 2 tbsp. lemon juice
- ¼ cup cranberry juice
- 1 cinnamon stick (3 inches)

- ½ tsp. whole cloves

Directions:

1. Start by tying all the whole spices in cheesecloth.

2. Now place the tied spices along with all other ingredients into the Crock-Pot.

3. Cover its lid and cook for 3 hours on a low setting.

4. Once done, remove its lid of the Crock-Pot carefully.

5. Strain the slow-cooked tea into the serving glasses.

6. Serve warm.

Nutrition:

- Calories: 158

- Total Fat: 35.2 g

- Saturated Fat: 15.2 g

- Cholesterol: 69 mg

- Sodium: 178 mg

- Total Carbs: 7.4 g

- Sugar: 1.1 g

- Fiber: 3.5 g

- Protein: 5.5 g

Wrapped Avocado Sticks

Preparation Time: 15 minutes

Cooking Time: 2 hours

Servings: 7

Ingredients:

- 5 oz. bacon, sliced
- 1 avocado, pitted
- 1 tsp. paprika
- ½ tsp. salt
- 2 tbsp. butter

Directions:

1. Cut the avocado into the medium sticks.
2. Sprinkle the avocado sticks with the paprika and salt.
3. Wrap the avocado sticks in the sliced bacon.
4. Place the avocado sticks in the slow cooker and add the butter.
5. Close the lid and cook the snack for 2 hours on High.
6. Cool the cooked avocado sticks to room temperature and serve!

Nutrition:

- Calories: 198
- Fat: 17.4
- Fiber: 2

- Carbs: 2.9

- Fiber: 1 g

- Protein: 8.1

Beef Recipes

Beef Ragout with Beans

Preparation Time: 10 minutes

Cooking Time: 5 hours

Servings: 5

Ingredients:

- 1 tbsp. tomato paste
- 1 cup mung beans, canned
- 1 carrot, grated
- 1 lb. beef stew meat, chopped
- 1 tsp. ground black pepper
- 2 cups water

Directions:

1. Pour water into the slow cooker.
2. Add meat, ground black pepper, and carrot.
3. Cook the mixture on High for 4 hours.
4. Then add tomato paste and mung beans. Stir the meal and cook it on high for 1 hour more.

Nutrition:

- Calories: 321
- Fat: 6 g
- Carbs: 18 g
- Sugar: 1.2 g
- Fiber: 1.5 g
- Sodium: 35 mg
- Protein: 30 g

Braised Beef

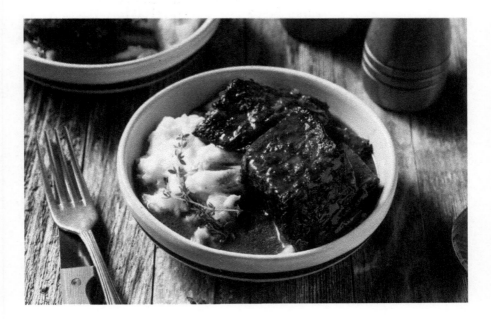

Preparation Time: 8 minutes

Cooking Time: 9 hours

Servings: 2

Ingredients:

- 8 oz. beef tenderloin, chopped
- 1 garlic clove, peeled
- 1 tsp. peppercorn
- 1 tsp. salt
- 1 tbsp. dried basil
- 2 cups water

Directions:

1. Put all ingredients from the list above in the slow cooker.

2. Gently stir the mixture and close the lid.

3. Cook the beef on low for 9 hours.

Nutrition:

- Calories: 233
- Fat: 18 g
- Carbs: 12 g
- Sugar: 1.2 g
- Fiber: 1.5 g
- Sodium: 35 mg
- Protein: 28 g

Coconut Beef

Preparation Time: 10 minutes

Cooking Time: 8 hours

Servings: 5

Ingredients:

- 1 cup baby spinach, chopped
- 1 cup coconut milk
- 1-lb. beef tenderloin, chopped
- 1 tsp. avocado oil
- 1 tsp. dried rosemary
- 1 tsp. garlic powder

Directions:

1. Roast meat in the avocado oil for 1 minute per side on high heat.
2. Ten transfer the meat in the slow cooker.
3. Add garlic powder, dried rosemary, coconut milk, and baby spinach.
4. Close the lid and cook the meal on Low for 8 hours.

Nutrition:

- Calories: 303
- Fat: 19 g
- Carbs: 3 g
- Sugar: 1.2 g

- Fiber: 1.5 g

- Sodium: 35 mg

- Protein: 26 g

Tasty Spiced Chili Beef Eye Roast

Preparation Time: 15 minutes

Cooking Time: 8 hours

Servings: 4

Ingredients:

- 3 lb. lean ground beef eye roast
- 2 tbsp. Worcestershire sauce
- 4 tbsp. fresh lime juice
- 1 ½ cups diced onions
- 1 cup diced red bell pepper
- 3 cloves minced garlic
- 3 minced and seeded Serrano chilies
- Salt and pepper
- ½ cup beef broth
- 1 cup canned tomatoes, diced
- ½ tsp. dried oregano

Directions:

1. Use salt and pepper to season the beef and put it into the slow cooker.
2. In a large bowl, whisk the remaining ingredients together and pour them over the beef.
3. Cook on low for 8 hours.
4. Use 2 forks to shred the beef.

Nutrition:

- Calories: 247
- Fat: 6 g
- Carbs: 13 g
- Sugar: 1.2 g
- Fiber: 1.5 g
- Sodium: 35 mg
- Protein: 21 g

Lamb & Pork

Root Beer Pulled Pork Sandwich

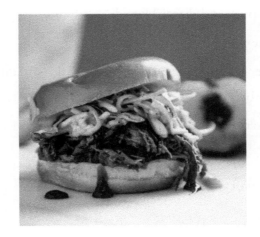

Preparation Time: 10 minutes

Cooking Time: 7 hours

Servings: 4

Ingredients:

- 1-2 cans root beer soda

- 2 cups BBQ sauce, plus some more for serving

- 2 pork loins, about 1 – 1 ½ lb.

- Salt and Pepper

- ½ cup prepared slaw

- 4 rolls

Directions:

1. Season the pork loins with pepper and salt.

2. Place pork in a slow cooker, and pour enough root beer and BBQ sauce to almost cover it.

3. Cook on low for 7-8 hours.

4. Remove pork and discard liquid.

5. Shred the pork.

6. To serve, warm the sandwich rolls. Add shredded pork with some barbecue sauce. Top with slaw.

7. Serve warm.

Nutrition:

- Calories: 446
- Fat: 18 g
- Carbs: 45 g
- Sugar: 1.2 g
- Fiber: 1.5 g
- Sodium: 35 mg
- Protein: 21 g

Smoky Baby Back Ribs

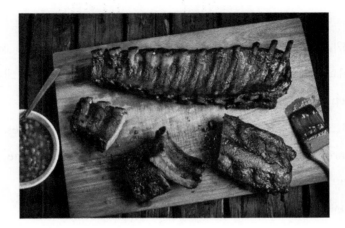

Preparation Time: 10 minutes

Cooking Time: 8 hours

Servings: 4

Ingredients:

- 2 baby back pork ribs racks, halved

- 1 cup barbecue sauce

- 1 tsp. liquid smoke (optional)

- 4 tbsp. barbecue spices mix

- Cooking spray

Directions:

1. Remove the membrane and excess fat from the ribs.

2. Rub each rib half rack with 1 tbsp. of the barbecue spice mix.

3. Spray slow cooker with cooking spray.

4. Place pork ribs in a slow cooker.

5. Combine the barbecue sauce and liquid smoke. Brush the racks lightly with half of the liquid smoke and barbecue sauce mix.

6. Cook on high for 5 hours until tender.

7. When ready to serve, remove ribs from the slow cooker, and place them on a foil-lined baking dish. Brush ribs with remaining barbecue sauce.

8. Broil the ribs in the oven for about 5-10 minutes. Watch carefully so they don't burn. This can also be done on the barbecue grill.

9. Serve warm with your favorite side dishes.

Nutrition:

- Calories: 432
- Fat: 16 g
- Carbs: 43 g
- Sugar: 1.2 g
- Fiber: 1.5 g
- Sodium: 35 mg
- Protein: 22 g

Sour and Sweet Meatballs

Preparation Time: 10 minutes

Cooking Time: 4 hours

Servings: 4

Ingredients:

- 16 pork meatballs, precooked
- ½ cup sugar
- 2 tbsp. cornstarch
- ⅓ Cup white vinegar
- 1 tbsp. soy sauce
- ½ tsp. chili garlic sauce
- 1 tsp. sesame oil
- ½ green pepper, diced
- 1 can pineapple chunks
- Cooked rice, for serving

Directions:

1. Place the meatballs in a slow cooker.
2. In a mixing bowl, whisk together the sugar, cornstarch, vinegar, soy sauce, chili garlic sauce, and sesame oil. Mix all together and pour over the meatballs.
3. Add the green pepper.
4. Cover, and cook for 4–4 ½ hours on LOW.
5. Add the pineapple and cook for 30 minutes more.

6. Serve over hot rice.

Nutrition:

- Calories: 476
- Fat: 29 g
- Carbs: 22 g
- Sugar: 1.2 g
- Fiber: 1.5 g
- Sodium: 35 mg
- Protein: 29 g

Amazing Pulled Pork

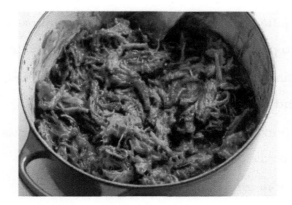

Preparation Time: 10 minutes

Cooking Time: 8 hours

Servings: 8

Ingredients:

- 5 lb. pork shoulder
- 2 tbsp. mustard
- 2 cups tomato purée
- 6 Medrol Dates, pitted
- ½ tsp. cloves, ground
- ½ tsp. cinnamon
- 2 tsps. salt
- Extra virgin olive oil
- Tortilla Wraps
- 8 eggs
- 1 tbsp. coconut flour

- ½ tsp. salt

Directions:

1. Place pitted dates in a blender, and mix until paste forms, add tomato purée, cinnamon, salt, black pepper, and mix.

2. Combine mustard, blended tomato puree, cloves, cinnamon, salt, and mix.

3. Place pork shoulder in the slow cooker, pour the sauce into the slow cooker, and coat pork shoulder.

4. Cook pork for 8 hours on high.

5. Once the pork is cooked, use a fork to shred.

6. For tortilla wraps, whisk eggs, add milk and flour, and mix until well combined.

7. Heat 4 tbsp. oil in a skillet on medium-high.

8. **Pour ⅛ of the mixture into the skillet and cook each side for 30 seconds.**

9. Spoon pork mixture into egg tortilla and serve.

Nutrition:

- Energy (calories): 928 kcal
- Protein: 81.13 g
- Fat: 60.37 g
- Carbohydrates: 9.89 g
- Fiber 1.3 g
- Sugars I5.29 g

Poultry & Chicken

Rotisserie Chicken

Preparation Time: 10 minutes

Cooking Time: 8 hours 5 minutes

Servings: 10

Ingredients:

- 1 organic whole chicken
- 1 tbsp. olive oil
- 1 tsp. thyme
- 1 tsp. rosemary
- 1 tsp. garlic, granulated
- Salt and pepper

Directions:

1. Start by seasoning the chicken with all the herbs and spices.
2. Broil this seasoned chicken for 5 minutes in the oven until golden brown.
3. Place this chicken in the Crock-Pot.
4. Cover it and cook for 8 hours on a low setting.
5. Serve warm.

Nutrition:

- Calories: 301
- Total Fat: 12.2 g
- Saturated Fat: 2.4 g
- Cholesterol: 110 mg
- Total Carbs: 2.5 g
- Fiber: 0.9 g
- Sugar: 1.4 g
- Sodium: 276 mg
- Potassium: 231 mg
- Protein: 28.8 g

Crock-Pot Chicken Adobo

Preparation Time: 10 minutes

Cooking Time: 8 hours

Servings: 6

Ingredients:

- ¼ cup apple cider vinegar
- 12 chicken drumsticks
- 1 onion, diced into slices
- 2 tbsp. olive oil
- 10 cloves garlic, smashed
- 1 cup gluten-free tamari
- ¼ cup diced green onion

Directions:

1. Place the drumsticks in the Crock-Pot and then add the remaining ingredients on top.
2. Cover it and cook for 8 hours on a low setting.
3. Mix gently, then serve warm.

Nutrition:

- Calories: 249
- Total Fat: 11.9 g
- Saturated Fat: 1.7 g
- Cholesterol: 78 mg

- Total Carbs: 1.8 g

- Fiber: 1.1 g

- Sugar: 0.3 g

- Sodium: 79 mg

- Potassium: 131 mg

- Protein: 25 g

Chicken Ginger Curry

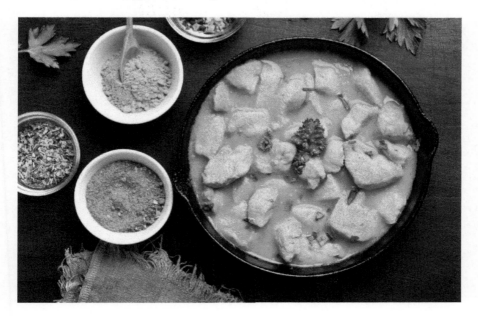

Preparation Time: 10 minutes

Cooking Time: 6 hours

Servings: 4

Ingredients:

- 1 ½ lb. chicken drumsticks (approx. 5 drumsticks) skin removed

- 1 (13.5 oz.) can coconut milk

- 1 onion, diced

- 4 cloves garlic, minced

- 1-inch knob fresh ginger, minced

- 1 Serrano pepper, minced

- 1 tbsp. Garam Masala

- ½ tsp. cayenne

- ½ tsp. paprika

- ½ tsp. turmeric

- salt and pepper, adjust to taste

Directions:

1. Start by throwing all the ingredients into the Crock-Pot.

2. Cover it and cook for 6 hours on a low setting.

3. Garnish as desired.

4. Serve warm.

Nutrition:

- Calories: 248

- Total Fat: 15.7 g

- Saturated Fat: 2.7 g

- Cholesterol: 75 mg

- Total Carbs: 8.4 g

- Fiber: 0g

- Sugar: 1.1 g

- Sodium: 94 mg

- Potassium: 331 mg

- Protein: 14.1 g

Thai Chicken Curry

Preparation Time: 10 minutes

Cooking Time: 2.5 hours

Servings: 2

Ingredients:

- 1 can coconut milk
- ½ cup chicken stock
- 1 lb. boneless, skinless chicken thighs, diced
- 1 2 tbsp. red curry paste
- 1 tbsp. coconut aminos
- 1 tbsp. fish sauce
- 2 3 garlic cloves, minced
- Salt and black pepper to taste
- red pepper flakes as desired
- 1 bag frozen mixed veggies

Directions:

1. Start by throwing all the ingredients except vegetables into the Crock-Pot.
2. Cover it and cook for 2 hours on a low setting.
3. Remove its lid and thawed veggies.
4. Cover the Crock-Pot again then continue cooking for another 30 minutes on a low setting.
5. Garnish as desired.

6. Serve warm.

Nutrition:

- Calories: 327
- Total Fat: 3.5 g
- Saturated Fat: 0.5 g
- Cholesterol: 162 mg
- Total Carbs: 56g
- Fiber: 0.4 g
- Sugar: 0.5 g
- Sodium: 142 mg
- Potassium: 558 mg
- Protein: 21.5 g

Fish & Seafood

Shrimp Tomato Medley

Preparation Time: 10 minutes

Cooking Time: 1 hour

Servings: 8

Ingredients:

- ½ tbsp. chili oil
- 4 scallions, diced
- 1½ tbsp. coconut oil
- 1 small ginger root, diced
- 8 cups chicken stock
- ¼ cup coconut aminos
- ¼ tsp. fish sauce
- 1 lb. shrimp, peeled and deveined
- ½ lb. tomatoes
- Black pepper ground, to taste
- 1 tbsp. sesame oil
- 1 (5 oz.) can bamboo shoots, sliced

Directions:

1. Start by throwing all the ingredients into your Crock-Pot.

2. Cover its lid and cook for 1 hour on a low setting.

3. Once done, remove its lid and stir it.

4. Serve warm.

Nutrition:

- Calories: 371

- Total Fat: 3.7 g

- Saturated Fat: 2.7 g

- Cholesterol: 168 mg

- Sodium: 121 mg

- Total Carbs: 4 g

- Fiber: 1.5 g

- Sugar: 0.3 g

- Protein: 26.5 g

Butter Glazed Mussels

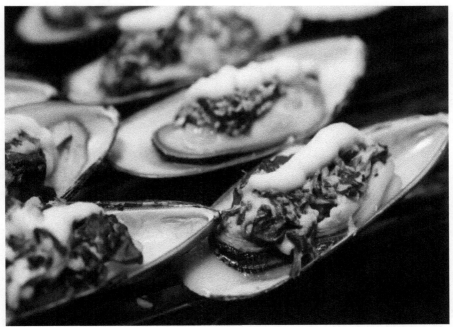

Preparation Time: 10 minutes

Cooking Time: 2 hours

Servings: 6

Ingredients:

- 1 tbsp. butter

- A splash lemon juice

- 2 lb. mussels, stripped and washed

- 2 garlic cloves, peeled and minced

Directions:

1. Start by throwing all the ingredients into your Crock-Pot.

2. Cover its lid and cook for 2 hours on a high setting.

3. Once done, remove its lid and stir it.

4. Serve warm.

Nutrition:

- Calories: 266

- Total Fat: 26.4 g

- Saturated Fat: 4 g

- Cholesterol: 13 mg

- Sodium: 455 mg

- Total Carbs: 5.4 g

- Sugar: 2 g

- Fiber: 1.6 g

- Protein: 20.6 g

Citrus Rich Octopus Salad

Preparation Time: 10 minutes

Cooking Time: 2 hours

Servings: 2

Ingredients:

- 3 oz. olive oil
- Juice 1 lemon
- 21 oz. octopus, rinsed
- 4 celery stalks, roughly diced
- Salt and black pepper ground, to taste
- 4 tbsp. fresh parsley, roughly diced

Directions:

1. Start by throwing all the ingredients into your Crock-Pot.
2. Cover its lid and cook for 2 hours on a low setting.
3. Once done, remove its lid and stir it.
4. Serve warm.

Nutrition:

- Calories: 225
- Total Fat: 17.7 g
- Saturated Fat: 3.2 g
- Cholesterol: 5 mg
- Sodium: 386 mg

- Total Carbs: 11.3 g
- Sugar: 7.1 g
- Fiber: 4.5 g
- Protein: 7.4 g

Creamy Clam Chowder Luncheon

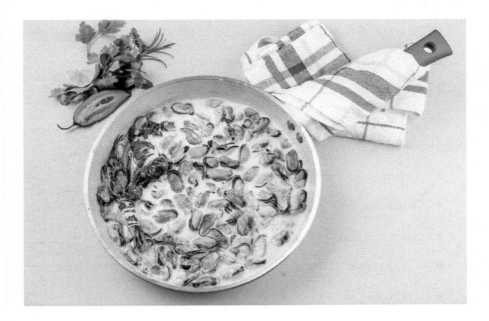

Preparation Time: 10 minutes

Cooking Time: 2 hours

Servings: 4

Ingredients:

- 2 cups chicken stock

- 1 tsp. ground thyme

- 14 oz. canned baby clams

- 1 cup celery stalks, roughly diced

- 2 cups heavy cream

- Salt and black pepper ground, to taste

- 1 cup onion, peeled and roughly diced

- 12 bacon strips, roughly diced

Directions:

1. Start by throwing all the ingredients into your Crock-Pot.

2. Cover its lid and cook for 2 hours on a high setting.

3. Once done, remove its lid and stir it.

4. Serve warm.

Nutrition:

- Calories: 449

- Total Fat: 28.7 g

- Saturated Fat: 14.9 g

- Cholesterol: 163 mg

- Sodium: 744 mg

- Total Carbs: 8.4 g

- Sugar: 2.6 g

- Fiber: 1.9 g

- Protein: 39.3 g

Vegetarian

Slow-Cooker Curried Butternut Squash Soup

Preparation Time: 7 minutes

Cooking Time: 8 hours

Servings: 4

Ingredients:

- 1 medium cubed butternut squash
- 1 lb. chopped organic carrots
- 4 cups unsalted vegetable stock organic
- 1 tsp. curry powder
- 1 tsp. sea salt
- ½ tsp. garlic powder
- ½ tsp. Garam masala
- ½ tsp. cumin

Directions:

1. Add all ingredients to Crock-Pot and cook at low for eight hours. Then blend with two more cups of stock, and it's ready.

Nutrition:

- Calories: 164
- Fat: 0 g

- 1 tsp. cumin
- 1 tsp. turmeric
- 1 tsp. powdered garlic
- ½ tsp. salt
- 29 oz. puree tomatoes canned
- ½ can coconut milk
- 2 cups any rice (basmati, quinoa, and cauliflower)
- ½ cup coconut milk
- ½ tsp. crushed ginger

Directions:

1. Add everything to Crock-Pot other than coconut milk and cook at low for eight hours.
2. Add the milk just before serving it.

Nutrition:

- Calories: 278
- Fat: 2 g
- Carbs: 46 g
- Sugar: 1.7 g
- Fiber: 5.2 g
- Sodium: 58 mg
- Protein: 16 g

Slow Cooker Vegetable Frittata (Low-Carb)

Preparation Time: 5 minutes

Cooking Time: 2 hours

Servings: 4

Ingredients:

- 6 eggs
- ½ cup of cheese
- 1 tbsp. of Parmesan cheese
- 4 oz. sliced mushrooms
- ¼ cup chopped fresh spinach
- 2 tsp. of Italian seasoning
- ¼ cup sliced cherry tomatoes
- 2 sliced green onions
- 1 tsp. of ghee

Directions:

1. Grease the Crock-Pot.
2. Add ghee to the pan and sauté vegetables. Transfer them to the Crock-Pot
3. Make an egg mix with seasonings and cheese.
4. Pour over the vegetables and cook at high for two hours.

Nutrition:

- Calories: 190
- Fat: 13 g

- Sugar: 1.7 g
- Fiber: 5.2 g
- Sodium: 58 mg
- Carbs: 3 g
- Protein: 14 g

Slow Cooker Eggplant Lasagna

Preparation Time: 35 minutes

Cooking Time: 2 hours

Servings: 4

Ingredients:

- Noodles 2 eggplant
- 1 diced onion,
- 1 diced bell pepper
- 1 cup cottage cheese
- 8 oz. mozzarella cheese
- 12 oz. pasta sauce

Directions:

1. Put eggplant noodles at the base and layer mozzarella and cottage cheese, sauce, onion, and peppers.
2. Repeat the layers three times and cook at high for two hours.
3. Serve hot.

Nutrition:

- Calories: 212
- Fat: 5 g
- Carbs: 16 g
- Sugar: 1.7 g
- Fiber: 5.2 g
- Sodium: 58 mg
- Protein: 14 g

Vegan & Vegetarian

Mushroom Risotto

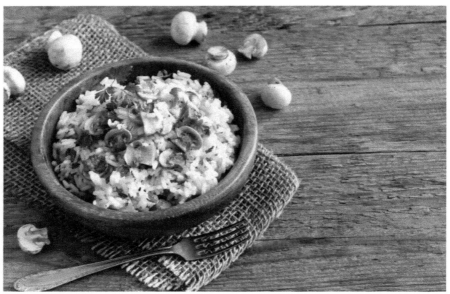

Preparation Time: 15 minutes

Cooking Time: 4 hours

Servings: 4

Ingredients:

- ¼ cup vegetable broth

- 1 lb. sliced Portobello mushrooms

- 1 lb. sliced white mushrooms
- ⅓ cup grated parmesan cheese
- 2 diced shallots
- 3 tbsp. chopped chives
- 3 tbsp. coconut oil
- 4 ½ cup rice cauliflower
- 4 tbsp. butter

Directions:

1. Heat-up oil and sauté mushrooms for 3 minutes till soft. Discard the liquid and set it to the side.
2. Add oil to skillet and sauté shallots 60 seconds.
3. Pour all recipe components into your pot and mix well to combine.
4. Cook for 3 hours on high heat. Serve topped with parmesan cheese.

Nutrition:

- Calories: 438
- Carbs: 5 g
- Fat: 17 g
- Sugar: 1.7 g
- Sodium: 58 mg
- Protein: 12 g

Vegan Bibimbap

Preparation Time: 15 minutes

Cooking Time: 45 minutes

Servings: 4

Ingredients:

- ½ cucumber, sliced into strips
- 1 grated carrot
- 1 sliced red bell pepper
- 1 tbsp. soy sauce
- 1 tsp. sesame oil
- 10 oz. riced cauliflower
- 2 tbsp. rice vinegar
- 2 tbsp. sesame seeds
- 2 tbsp. Sriracha sauce
- 4-5 broccoli florets
- 7 oz. tempeh, sliced into squares
- Liquid sweetener

Directions:

1. In a bowl, combine tempeh squares with 1 tbsp. soy sauce and 2 tbsp. vinegar. Set aside to soak. Slice veggies.
2. Add carrot, broccoli, and peppers to the slow cooker. Cook on high for 30 minutes.
3. Add cauliflower rice to the slow cooker; cook for 5 minutes.

4. Add sweetener, oil, soy sauce, vinegar, and Sriracha to the slow cooker. Don't hesitate to add a bit of water if you find the mixture to be too thick.

Nutrition:

- Calories: 119
- Carbs: 0 g
- Fat: 18 g
- Sugar: 1.7 g
- Sodium: 58 mg
- Protein: 8 g

Avocado Pesto Kelp Noodles

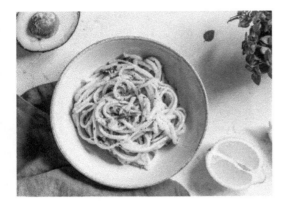

Preparation Time: 15 minutes

Cooking Time: 1 hour & 30 minutes

Servings: 2

Ingredients:

Pesto:

- ¼ cup basil
- ½ cup extra-virgin olive oil
- 1 avocado
- 1 cup baby spinach leaves
- 1 tsp. salt
- 1-2 garlic cloves
- 1 package kelp noodles

Directions:

1. Add kelp noodles to the slow cooker with just enough water to cover them. Cook on high for 45-60 minutes.

2. In the meantime, combine pesto ingredients in a blender, blending till smooth and incorporated.

3. Stir in pesto and heat noodle mixture for 10 minutes.

Nutrition:

- Calories: 321
- Carbs: 1 g
- Fat: 32 g
- Sugar: 1.7 g
- Sodium: 58 mg
- Protein: 2 g

Vegan Cream of Mushroom Soup

Preparation Time: 15 minutes

Cooking Time: 1 hour & 40 minutes

Servings: 2

Ingredients:

- ¼ tsp. sea salt
- ½ diced yellow onion
- ½ tsp. extra-virgin olive oil
- 1 ½ cup chopped white mushrooms
- **1 ⅔ cup unsweetened almond milk**
- 1 tsp. onion powder
- 2 cup cauliflower florets

Directions:

1. Add cauliflower, pepper, salt, onion powder, and milk to the slow cooker. Stir and set to cook on high for 1 hour.

2. With olive oil, sauté onions and mushrooms together for 8 to 10 minutes till softened.

3. Allow the cauliflower mixture to cool off a bit and add to the blender. Blend until smooth. Then blend in mushroom mixture.

4. Pour back into the slow cooker and heat for 30 minutes.

Nutrition:

- Calories: 281
- Carbs: 3 g
- Fat: 16 g
- Sugar: 1.7 g
- Sodium: 58 mg
- Protein: 11 g

Soups, Chilis & Stew

Keto/Low Carb Unstuffed Cabbage Roll

Preparation Time: 10 minutes

Cooking Time: 6 hours

Servings: 9

Ingredients:

- ½ diced small onion
- 2 minced garlic cloves
- 1 ½ lbs. minced beef
- 3 cups of beef broth
- 14 oz. diced tomatoes can
- 8 oz. tomato sauce can
- ¼ cup Bragg's Aminos
- 1 chopped cabbage
- 3 tsp. of Worcestershire Sauce
- ½ tsp. of parsley
- ½ tsp. of salt
- ½ tsp. of pepper

Directions:

1. Turn the ground beef brown with garlic and onion and drain afterward.

2. Place all ingredients in the Crock-Pot and cover.

3.   Using high temperature, cook for 3 hours.

Nutrition:

- Calories: 217
- Fat: 16 g
- Carbs: 6 g
- Sugar: 1.7 g
- Sodium: 58 mg
- Protein: 15 g

Bacon Cheeseburger Soup

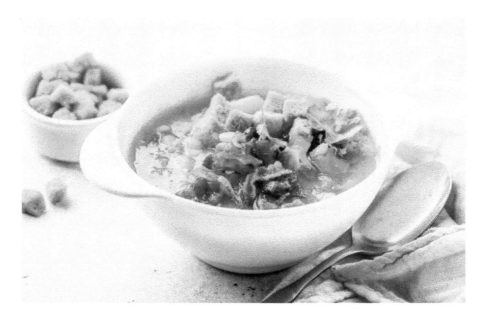

Preparation Time: 15 minutes

Cooking Time: 8 hours

Servings: 6

Ingredients:

- 5 bacon slices

- 1 lb. minced beef

- 2 tsp. spices seasoning

- 1 clove minced garlic

- ½ cup diced onion

- ½ cup diced green pepper,

- 1 cup chopped cauliflower,

- ½ cup diced carrot,

- 1 cup diced celery,

- 4 cups chicken broth

- 1 cup heavy cream

- ¼ tsp. xanthan gum

- 1 cup cheddar cheese shredded

Directions:

1. Prepare ground beef and bacon as usual.

2. Insert celery, bacon, beef, carrots, and broth into the cooker.

3. At low temperature, cook for 8 hours.

4. Whish heavy cream in xanthan gum.

5. Carry to boil and low the heat.

6. Transfer to the soup and mix.

7. Place ¼ cup of cheese in one time and mix.

8. Cover with a lid and allow it to cook for 20 more minutes.

Nutrition:

- Calories: 452

- Fat: 21 g

- Sugar: 1.7 g

- Sodium: 58 mg

- Carbs: 4 g

- Protein: 28 g

Keto Jalapeno Popper Soup

Preparation Time: 5 minutes

Cooking Time: 4 hours

Servings: 4

Ingredients:

- 4 bacon slices
- 2 tbsp. butter
- ½ medium diced onion
- ¼ cup chopped pickled jalapenos
- 2 cups of chicken broth
- 2 cups shredded chicken cooked
- 4 oz. cream cheese
- ⅓ cup of heavy cream
- 1 cup sharp cheddar shredded
- ¼ tsp. garlic powder
- Salt & Pepper

Directions:

1. Add the prepared bacon with the rest of the ingredients.
2. Place heavy cream and cheddar separately.
3. Cook for 4 hours over low settings.
4. Add cream and cheddar while serving.

Nutrition:

- Calories: 446
- Fat: 35 g
- Carbs: 4 g
- Sugar: 1.7 g
- Sodium: 58 mg
- Protein: 28 g

Crock-Pot Low Carb Taco Soup

Preparation Time: 10 minutes

Cooking Time: 2 hours

Servings: 7

Ingredients:

- 2 lbs. minced beef cooked
- 2 tbsp. minced garlic
- 2 tbsp. taco seasoning
- 10 oz. diced tomatoes Rotel
- 4 oz. diced canned green chilis
- 8 oz. cream cheese
- 4 cups of beef broth
- ½ tsp. chili powder
- ⅔ cup of onion

Directions:

1. Prepare the ground beef.
2. Add the ground beef to the Crock-Pot after spraying with no-stick spray.
3. Add cream cheese to the Crock-Pot.
4. Then add the diced onions.
5. Place Rotel, chili powder, garlic, green chilis, and beef broth.

6. Cover with lid and allow it to cook for 2 hours at high temperature.

Nutrition:

- Calories: 369
- Fat: 24 g
- Carbs: 6 g
- Sugar: 1.7 g
- Sodium: 58 mg
- Protein: 30 g

Side Dishes

Creamy Green Beans

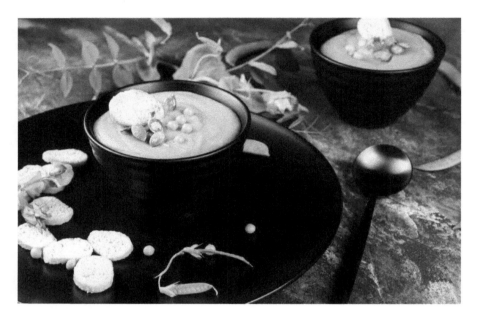

Preparation Time: 10 minutes

Cooking Time: 2 hours

Servings: 4

Ingredients:

- 2 cups green beans, trimmed and halved

- 1 tbsp. tahini paste

- 1 tsp. turmeric powder

- 1 red chili, minced
- ½ tsp. salt
- 1 tsp. olive oil
- ⅓ cup heavy cream

Directions:

1. Put green beans in the slow cooker.

2. Add the rest of the ingredients and put the lid on.

3. Cook the mix for 2 hours on High.

4. Put in the serving bowls.

Nutrition:

- Calories: 134
- Fat: 5.9 g
- Fiber: 3.1 g
- Carbs: 6.3 g
- Sugar: 1.7 g
- Sodium: 58 mg
- Protein: 6.7 g

Artichoke and Broccoli Mix

Preparation Time: 10 minutes

Cooking Time: 5 hours

Servings: 4

Ingredients:

- 4 tbsp. lemon juice

- 2 artichokes, trimmed and halved

- 1 cup broccoli florets

- 1 tsp. tahini paste

- ½ tsp. sweet paprika

- 3 tbsp. olive oil

- ½ tsp. salt

- ½ garlic clove, minced

- ¼ cup water

Directions:

1. In the slow cooker, mix the artichokes with the broccoli and the other ingredients and close the lid.

2. Cook the vegetable for 5 hours on low.

3. Divide between plates and serve.

Nutrition:

- Calories: 142

- Fat: 11.2 g

- Fiber: 4.6 g
- Carbs: 9.5 g
- Sugar: 1.7 g
- Sodium: 58 mg
- Protein: 3 g

Collard Greens and Mushrooms

Preparation Time: 10 minutes

Cooking Time: 3.5 hours

Servings: 4

Ingredients:

- 9 oz. collard greens, trimmed, chopped

- 2 spring onions, chopped

- 1 cup white mushrooms, sliced

- 1 cup water

- 1 tsp. salt

- 1 tsp. chili powder

- 1 tsp. olive oil

Directions:

1. In the slow cooker, mix the greens with mushrooms and the other ingredients and close the slow cooker lid.

2. Cook the greens for 3.5 hours on high.

3. Divide into bowls and serve.

Nutrition:

- Calories: 184

- Fat: 7.5 g

- Fiber: 4.8 g

- Carbs: 7.6 g

- Sugar: 1.7 g

- Sodium: 58 mg

- Protein: 5.8 g

Lime Zucchini Noodles

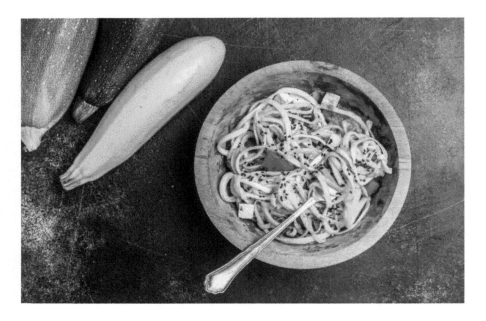

Preparation Time: 10 minutes

Cooking Time: 1 hour and 30 minutes

Servings: 4

Ingredients:

- 7 oz. zucchini noodles
- 1 tbsp. balsamic vinegar
- 1 tbsp. lime juice
- ¼ tsp. sweet paprika
- ½ tsp. salt
- ⅓ cup water
- 1 tsp. butter

Directions:

1. In the slow cooker, mix the noodles with the vinegar and the other ingredients.

2. Put the lid on and cook noodles for 1.5 hours on low.

3. Divide between plates and serve.

Nutrition:

- Calories: 120
- Fat: 5.1 g
- Fiber: 5.3 g
- Carbs: 0.1 g
- Sugar: 1.7 g
- Sodium: 58 mg
- Protein: 3.4 g

Desserts

Chocolate Pecan Cake

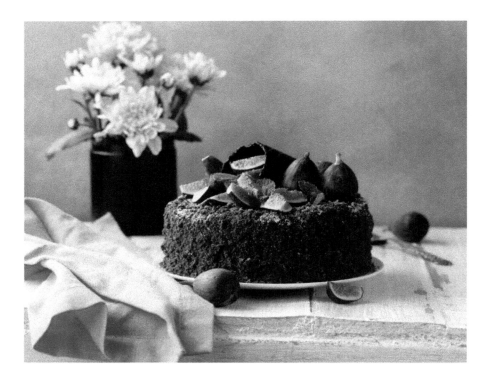

Preparation Time: 10 minutes

Cooking Time: 5 hours

Servings: 4

Ingredients:

- 1 cup coconut flour
- ⅓ cup almond butter, melted

- ¼ cup water
- 1 tsp. almond extract
- 2 tbsp. Stevia
- 1 tsp. baking powder
- ½ oz. dark chocolate, chopped
- 3 eggs, beaten
- 2 pecans, chopped
- Cooking spray

Directions:

1. In a bowl mix the coconut flour with almond butter water and the other ingredients except for the cooking spray.
2. Spray the slow cooker with cooking spray from inside and pour the cake mixture.
3. Flatten the surface of the cake mixture well and close the lid.
4. Cook the spoon cake for 5 hours on low.

Nutrition:

- Calories: 180
- Fat: 4.6 g
- Fiber: 2 g
- Sugar: 11.7 g
- Sodium: 58 mg
- Carbs: 7.2 g
- Protein: 4.3 g

Lemon Scones

Preparation Time: 15 minutes

Cooking Time: 2.5 hours

Servings: 6

Ingredients:

- 2 cups almond flour
- ½ cup coconut oil
- 2 tbsp. lemon juice
- 1 tsp. cinnamon powder
- 1 tsp. baking powder
- 1 egg, beaten
- 4 tbsp. Swerve

Directions:

1. In the mixing bowl, combine the flour with the coconut oil and the other ingredients and stir well.
2. Line the slow cooker with baking paper.
3. Make the ball from the dough and place it in the slow cooker.
4. Cut the dough into 6 scones and close the lid.
5. Cook the scones for 2.5 hours on high.
6. Then chill the cooked dessert well and cut the dough into scones again.

Nutrition:

- Calories: 221
- Fat: 14.4 g
- Fiber: 1 g
- Carbs: 6.6 g
- Sugar: 11.7 g
- Sodium: 58 mg
- Protein: 3.1 g

Strawberries Cake

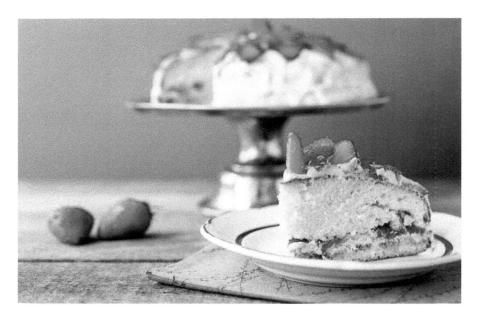

Preparation Time: 15 minutes

Cooking Time: 4.5 hours

Servings: 4

Ingredients:

- ⅓ cup strawberries, chopped
- 1 cup coconut flour
- ¼ cup butter, softened
- ¾ cup stevia
- 1 tsp. vanilla extract
- ¾ tsp. cinnamon powder

- 1 tsp. coconut oil

Directions:

1. Spread the slow cooker bottom with coconut oil.

2. Place the chopped strawberries in the slow cooker and flatten them to get the layer shape.

3. In a bowl mix the rest of the ingredients, stir and knead the dough a bit.

4. Then place the dough over the strawberries. Flatten it well and close the lid.

5. Cook the cake for 4.5 hours on low.

6. When the cake is cooked, transfer it to the serving plates and eat hot.

Nutrition:

- Calories: 160
- Fat: 16.2 g
- Fiber: 1.1 g
- Carbs: 3.2 g
- Sugar: 11.7 g
- Sodium: 58 mg
- Protein: 1.7 g

Almond Roll

Preparation Time: 15 minutes

Cooking Time: 3.5 hours

Servings: 6

Ingredients:

- 1 tsp. baking powder
- 1 cup almond flour
- 1 tbsp. ground cinnamon
- 2 tbsp. stevia
- ⅓ cup coconut oil
- 1 tsp. almond extract
- 1 egg, beaten
- ¾ cup Mascarpone cream

Directions:

1. In a bowl mix the flour with coconut oil and the other ingredients except for the cinnamon and stevia.
2. Mix up together ground cinnamon with stevia
3. Roll up the dough with the help of the rolling pin.
4. Spread the surface of the dough with ground cinnamon mixture and roll it into the log.
5. Cut the log into 6 buns and secure the edges of every bun.
6. Line the Crock-Pot with baking paper.
7. Place the buns in the Crock-Pot and close the lid.

8. Cook the cinnamon roll for 3.5 hours on high.

9. Check if the rolls are cooked with the help of the toothpick – if it is dry, the buns are cooked.

10. Chill the dessert well and then remove from the Crock-Pot in the serving plate.

Nutrition:

- Calories: 208
- Sugar: 11.7 g
- Sodium: 58 mg
- Fat: 15.3 g
- Fiber: 1.1 g
- Carbs: 8.2 g
- Protein: 4.2 g

Measurement Conversion Chart

Volume Equivalents (Liquid)

US STANDARD	US STANDARD (oz.)	METRIC (APPROXIMATE)
2 tbsp.	1 fl. oz.	30 mL
¼ cup	2 fl. oz.	60 mL
½ cup	4 fl. oz.	120 mL
1 cup	8 fl. oz.	240 mL
1½ cups	12 fl. oz.	355 mL
2 cups or 1 pint	16 fl. oz.	475 mL
4 cups or 1 quart	32 fl. oz.	1 L
1 gallon	128 fl. oz.	4 L

Volume Equivalents (Dry)

US STANDARD	METRIC (APPROXIMATE)
¼ tsp.	1 mL
½ tsp.	2 mL
1 tsp.	5 mL
1 tbsp.	15 mL
¼ cup	59 mL
cup	79 mL
½ cup	118 mL
1 cup	177 mL

Oven Temperatures

FAHRENHEIT (F)	CELSIUS (C) (APPROXIMATE)
250°F	120 °C
300°F	150°C
325°F	165°C
350°F	180°C
375°F	190°C
400°F	200°C
425°F	220°C
450°F	230°C

Weight Equivalents

US STANDARD	METRIC (APPROXIMATE)
½ oz.	15 g
1 oz.	30 g
2 oz.	60 g
4 oz.	115 g
8 oz.	225 g
12 oz.	340 g
16 oz. or 1 lb.	455 g